CELLULITE

Uncovering Cellulite: A Look at What Causes and Affects Cellulite

CARL JUAN

Table of Contents

Introductory

Cellulite is the dimpled or lumpy look of skin, most noticeable on the thighs, buttocks, hips, and belly. It's a widespread aesthetic worry, especially among women. The lumpy appearance of cellulite results from the disproportional distribution of subcutaneous fat. It's not a disease or illness, but rather a cosmetic concern.

- Several factors, including heredity, hormone fluctuations, dietary and lifestyle decisions, and underlying connective tissue structure, have been linked to cellulite. Even while cellulite is not indicative of ill health, many people try to get rid of its look with treatments like massage, lotions, and even liposuction and laser therapy. Results from these treatments, if they work at all, tend to be short-lived and inconsistent.

• Even though a healthy lifestyle—including regular exercise, a balanced diet, and plenty of water—may not completely erase cellulite, it can help lessen its appearance. Expectations for the treatment and management of cellulite should be reasonable given its prevalence and naturalness.

CHAPTER ONE

Cellulite: What You Need to Know

Knowing the nature of cellulite, its origins, and possible remedies is essential. The following are some of the most important facts about cellulite:

1. The dimpled or lumpy appearance of skin, especially on the thighs, buttocks, hips, and belly, is referred to as cellulite. It results from the uneven distribution of fat just below the skin's surface.

2. Causes:

• One's family history is a major contributor to whether or not they develop cellulite. You might have a higher risk of getting cellulite if other members of your family already have it.

• Changes in hormone levels, such as those experienced during pregnancy, adolescence, and menopause, have been linked to an increased likelihood of cellulite formation.

• Cellulite's visual impact may be influenced by the strength and organization of the connective tissues lying just below the skin. Fat may protrude due to weakened connective tissues, giving the appearance of dimples.

- Diet and Lifestyle: An poor diet, lack of exercise, and smoking might contribute to the development of cellulite. Its visibility might be diminished by keeping a healthy lifestyle.

3. Treatment:

- Topical Creams: Some creams and lotions claim to minimize the appearance of cellulite, although their effectiveness is frequently limited and short.

Cellulite and blood flow can both be temporarily improved with massage techniques like lymphatic drainage massage.

- Laser and Radiofrequency Therapies: The application of heat and energy in these procedures has been shown to increase collagen formation and reduce fat. They have the potential to reduce the visual impact of cellulite temporarily.

While liposuction can reduce the appearance of cellulite by eliminating fat cells, it is not a foolproof method of doing so.

- Reducing the appearance of cellulite and preventing its formation can be accomplished with a healthy lifestyle that includes eating a balanced diet, staying hydrated, engaging in regular exercise, and not smoking.

While treatments and alterations to one's lifestyle can help lessen cellulite's appearance, it's not always possible to get rid of it entirely. Cellulite is a normal part of aging, and while some treatments may help, the degree of improvement varies from person to person. The most practical method of combating cellulite is to manage one's expectations and prioritize one's health and well-being in general.

Contributing Factors to Cellulite

There isn't just one thing that causes cellulite; rather, a number of variables work together. Cellulite can be attributed to the following causes:

1. Genetics: Genetic predisposition can play a key influence in the development of cellulite. Your risk of developing cellulite may increase if other members of your family also have it.

2. Hormonal Changes: Hormonal variations in the body can lead to cellulite production. Cellulite may be exacerbated by the hormonal changes that occur during puberty, pregnancy, and menopause, particularly those involving estrogen.

3. The production of collagen, a protein that aids in skin firmness, declines with age, which causes the skin to lose its suppleness. Because of this, cellulite may stand out much more.

4. Cellulite can be affected by the structure of the connective tissues just below the skin. The dimpled appearance is caused by fat protruding through connective tissues that are weaker or less supportive.

5. Fat and Muscle: An Unhealthy Disproportion Between the Two Causes of Cellulite. Cellulite's visibility can be exacerbated by excess body fat pressing against the connective tissues, although strong, toned muscles can assist support the skin and mitigate this effect.

6. The appearance of cellulite can be exacerbated by poor dietary choices and an inactive lifestyle, both of which can lead to weight gain. These include an abundance of processed and high-sugar foods.

7. Cellulite may become more pronounced in those who smoke due to the negative effects of poor circulation and the weakened skin that results from smoking.

8.   Dehydration: Inadequate hydration can lead to decreased skin suppleness, making cellulite more apparent. Keeping your skin properly hydrated is crucial to its overall health.

9. Chronic stresses can alter your hormone levels, which may have a role in the appearance of cellulite.

Cellulite is a normal part of the aging process and should not be seen as a sign of bad health, as is a widespread misconception. While numerous treatments and lifestyle adjustments can help lessen the appearance of cellulite, total eradication is typically tough. The most efficient method of controlling and reducing cellulite's visibility is to take a comprehensive approach to health, which includes a balanced diet, frequent exercise, and a healthy lifestyle.

CHAPTER TWO
Skin Structure and Function

The skin is the largest organ in the body and has several critical roles, such as providing protection, regulating body temperature, providing feeling, and preventing dehydration. It's built up of different levels, and they all do different things. The epidermis, dermis, and subcutaneous tissue (hypodermis) are the main components of the skin.

1. The epidermis is the skin's outermost layer. It provides a physical barrier against the environment. Multiple layers make up this structure.

The stratum corneum is the outermost layer of skin and is made up of dead, keratin-filled keratinocytes. It's a shield from the elements that threaten our safety.

- **Stratum lucidum:** a thin, see-through layer present in thick skin regions like the palms and soles.

Granules of lipids and keratin are seen in the cells of the stratum granulosum. These lipids help waterproof the skin.

Spiny projections from cells in the o Stratum Spinosum contribute to immunological responses.

The epidermis's innermost layer, known as the stratum basale (or stratum germinativum), is where brand-new skin cells are created. Melanocytes are the cells responsible for skin color because they generate the pigment melanin.

2. The dermis is a deeper layer of skin that is composed of more substantial connective tissue than the epidermis.

- **Blood Vessels:** These bring oxygen and nutrients to the skin and aid in keeping the body at a constant temperature.

• **Hair Follicles:** Hair shafts grow from hair follicles in the dermis.

The perspiration produced by your sweat glands is a natural way to keep your body at a comfortable temperature.

The sebaceous glands produce sebum, a lubricating and protective oil for the skin.

Touch, pain, and temperature feeling are all senses that rely on sensory nerve endings, which are abundant in the dermis.

Fibers of collagen and elastin, found in the dermis, give the skin its strength, pliability, and resilience.

3. The hypodermis, or subcutaneous tissue, is the layer directly beneath the dermis. Insulation and cushioning are provided by the adipose (fat) tissue that makes up most of it. Additionally, this layer links the skin to the underlying fascia, muscles, and skeletal framework.

• The skin's layers of structure are only the beginning of its usefulness. It's essential forwarding against harm, maintaining a comfortable internal temperature (by perspiration and alterations in blood flow), and gathering sensory data from the surrounding environment. Vitamin D can also be produced by skin exposure to sunlight.

Maintaining a healthy lifestyle, including correct diet and protection from excessive sun exposure, is crucial to keep the skin functioning properly and looking its best, which is why it is so important to the general health of the body.

The skin is an intricate organ with many different parts and functions that are crucial to a person's well-being. It keeps the body at a comfortable temperature, protects us from harm, and aids in both sensation and communication. **The skin's structure and functions are summarized below.**

1. Epidermis:

- To begin, let's talk about the epidermis, the skin's outermost layer.

What It Does:

- This barrier prevents the entry of hazardous bacteria, damaging rays from the sun, and physical harm to the body.

- **Waterproofing:** The epidermis contains cells loaded with keratin, which helps prevent water loss from the body.

- Pigmentation is achieved through the production of melanin by melanocytes in the basal layer of the epidermis, which gives skin its color and protects it from the sun.

2. Dermis:

- Located beneath the outer layer of skin (the epidermis), the dermis is a complex network of connective tissues, blood vessels, and other components.

What It Does:

- **Support:** The dermis offers structural support to the skin.

Touch, pressure, pain, and temperature are all senses that are transmitted via the nerve endings found in this area.

- **Hair and Glands:** The dermis houses hair follicles, sweat glands, and sebaceous glands.

- **Blood Vessels:** Blood vessels in the dermis assist regulate body temperature by constricting or dilating to control blood flow to the skin.

Skin's strength, suppleness, and resilience come from the dermal fibers collagen and elastin.

3. Hypodermis (Under the Skin):

• Adipose (fat) tissue predominates in the subcutaneous layer, which lies beneath the dermis.

What It Does:

• Thermal insulation is provided, which aids in maintaining a healthy internal environment.

• Padding: Adipose tissue serves as a shock absorber, keeping vital organs and other tissues beneath it safe.

- **Fat Storage:** Excess calories are stored in this layer.

4. Anatomy Lesson: Hair, Nails, and Glandular Systems

Hair follicles, nail beds, and different glands of the skin:

Hair shafts develop inside of follicles in the skin.

Nails are made of keratin and serve to safeguard the fingers and toes.

The perspiration produced by your sweat glands aids in keeping you cool through evaporative cooling.

The sebaceous glands produce sebum, an oily material that keeps the skin and hair from drying out.

5. Sensation:

• The skin has many sensory receptors that send signals to the brain about things like touch, temperature, and pain.

6. Infection Resistance:

• Initiating immune responses and serving as a barrier against invading pathogens are both functions of the skin's role in the body's immune system.

7. Synthesis of Vitamin D:

• Vitamin D, necessary for bone health and other body processes, is synthesized by the skin in response to exposure to UVB light from the sun.

In summary, the skin is a multipurpose organ that performs vital responsibilities in protecting the body, regulating temperature, and promoting sensory experience. Taking care of your skin by using the right products, staying out of the sun, and living a healthy lifestyle is crucial to your overall health.

CHAPTER THREE
Explanation of Subcutaneous Fat

The layer of fat directly under the skin is called subcutaneous fat or subcutaneous adipose tissue (SAT). Visceral fat, which is stored in the abdominal cavity and around the internal organs, is the other main form of body fat. Subcutaneous fat is present throughout the body and varies in thickness depending on an individual's genetics, gender, age, and general body composition.

1. Subcutaneous fat is found everywhere beneath the skin. It shows up anywhere from the arms and legs to the buttocks and

stomach. Subcutaneous fat can be distributed in a variety of ways.

2. Subcutaneous fat is important for a number of reasons.

• Because it prevents heat from escaping the body, it helps maintain a comfortable internal temperature.

Subcutaneous fat stores extra calories as triglycerides, which the body can use when energy is low.

3. Subcutaneous fat thickness varies greatly from person to person. Factors that determine subcutaneous fat thickness include heredity, age, gender, hormone changes, and total body composition. Subcutaneous fat is more prevalent in women than in men.

4. Considerations of Appearance Subcutaneous fat is responsible for the sculpting and defining of the skin. However, too much subcutaneous fat might affect a person's risk for diseases like cellulite and their general physical look.

5. Health Implications: While some subcutaneous fat is important for insulation and energy storage, excess subcutaneous fat, especially in the stomach region, might be related with health concerns.

Obesity, insulin resistance, and an upped risk of cardiovascular disease have all been linked to excessive quantities of abdomen subcutaneous fat.

6. It is essential to differentiate between subcutaneous fat and visceral fat. Health concerns such as metabolic syndrome, type 2 diabetes, and heart disease are more strongly associated with visceral fat, which is the fat that surrounds internal organs in the abdominal cavity. However, subcutaneous fat has a lower metabolic rate and is therefore thought to provide less of a health concern.

7. Different people will have different amounts of subcutaneous fat and visceral fat distributed throughout their bodies. The amount and location of subcutaneous fat can be affected by lifestyle factors like regular exercise and a balanced diet.

Subcutaneous fat, or fat right under the skin, has several critical functions, including thermal regulation, energy storage, and aesthetics. Subcutaneous fat is a natural part of the human body, but too much of it, especially in some locations, can be problematic. Subcutaneous fat can be controlled and general health can be improved by adhering to a healthy lifestyle that includes frequent exercise and a balanced diet.

What Connective Tissue Does

Connective tissue is a diverse and critical component of the body that plays several important tasks in sustaining and linking various tissues and organs. It helps keep the body together, supports its mechanics, and allows for the exchange of information between various organs and tissues. Collagen, elastin, fibrous connective tissue, and other specialized structures are all part of connective tissue. Some of the most important things connective tissue does are the following:

• The structure and support for many different tissues and organs are provided by connective tissue. It aids in the upkeep of the body's form and structure. Tendons and ligaments, for instance, are two examples of thick regular connective tissue that serve to anchor muscles to bones and bones to other bones, respectively, in order to provide stability and ease of movement.

- Connective tissue may have a protective function. Bone tissue, which serves to shield internal organs and support the body, is an example of a specialized connective tissue.

- Oxygen, nutrition, hormones, and waste materials are all transported throughout the body by this connective tissue known as blood. It consists of blood cells suspended in a liquid extracellular matrix.

- Adipose tissue (also known as adipose) is a type of loose connective tissue that mostly stores energy as triglycerides. This power can be made available when called for.

• Insulation against heat loss: Adipose tissue also functions as an insulator, which aids in maintaining a healthy internal body temperature.

• Connective tissue provides protection from infection because it houses immune cells and helps the body mount an immunological response to harmful invaders. For example, lymphoid tissue, a form of loose connective tissue, contains immune cells important for battling infection.

• Connective tissue is essential for the transmission of electrical signals and for establishing two-way communication between different regions of the body, and this is especially true in the nervous system.

• Connective tissue plays an important role in the repair and healing of injured tissues. Fibroblasts are cells found in connective tissue that help produce extracellular matrix, which is used to patch up injured areas.

• Structure Preservation Connective tissue provides the stroma or structural framework in many organs, ensuring that their functional components remain in place. Connective tissue in the liver or kidneys, for instance, plays a role in supporting the structure of those organs.

• Cartilage is a type of connective tissue found in joints that serves to cushion the bones and absorb shock. Synovial fluid, a type of connective tissue, also serves to lubricate joint motion.

• Connective tissue aids in the production of scar tissue, which aids in the repair and stabilization of injured parts of the body, following injury.

Depending on its context and role in the body, connective tissue displays a wide range of unique properties and functions. Together, these roles ensure the body's structure, defense, and homeostasis remain intact and stable.

CHAPTER FOUR
Living Conditions and Cellulite

How much cellulite you have and how quickly it appears might be affected by your way of life. Adopting a healthy lifestyle can help minimize the appearance of cellulite and enhance the skin's health despite the fact that cellulite is influenced by a number of variables, including genetics and hormonal fluctuations. Some examples of how your daily habits may be contributing to that cellulite:

• Nutritional deficiencies can contribute to cellulite. High-sugar, high-fat, processed foods can cause weight gain and fat storage, both of which can exacerbate cellulite. A healthy diet that emphasizes full, nutrient-dense meals can aid with weight management and lessen the visibility of cellulite.

• Keeping yourself hydrated is crucial to maintaining healthy skin. By keeping the skin supple and hydrated, cellulite can be concealed. Consuming an adequate amount of water can help the body in several ways, including the removal of pollutants.

• **Exercise:** Regular physical activity can help minimize the appearance of cellulite by increasing muscle tone and circulation. By strengthening and conditioning the muscles beneath the skin, cardio and weight training can help reduce the appearance of cellulite. Exercising can lead to weight loss, which in turn may decrease the amount of fat cells that cause cellulite.

• Chemicals in tobacco and alcohol can dehydrate the skin and slow blood flow, both of which can accentuate the appearance of cellulite. The skin's elasticity and health can suffer from excessive alcohol use because of the body's tendency to dehydrate. Reducing or eliminating these practices can help overall skin health.

• The visibility of cellulite can be mitigated by keeping a healthy body composition, which involves a balance of muscle and body fat. Strength training can help you gain muscle, which can help your skin look more toned and younger.

• Chronic stress might alter your hormone levels, which may play a role in cellulite formation. Meditation and other stress-reduction practices can help lessen the severity of these side effects.

• **Clothes and Shoes**: Tight clothing and high heels can aggravate cellulite because they constrict blood flow and add pressure to specific parts of the body. Selecting loose-fitting garments and shoes may aid in mitigating these variables.

• **Skincare:** Taking care of your skin properly can improve its health and lessen the visibility of cellulite. Exfoliating and hydrating the skin on a regular basis can help it look and feel better.

It's worth noting that cellulite is a normal part of the aging process, so getting rid of it entirely can be challenging. Results from making adjustments to one's lifestyle, such as those intended to improve one's skin health, can differ from person to person. The presence of cellulite says nothing about your general health, either. So, rather than focusing just on cellulite, it's crucial to maintain a well-rounded, healthy lifestyle for general health and happiness.

Cellulite and Skincare

Skincare can play a part in improving the appearance of cellulite by enhancing general skin health and making the skin look more toned and smoother.

Although skincare products alone may not eradicate cellulite entirely, they can lessen its appearance. Listed below are some methods that could improve your skincare routine:

• With consistent exfoliation, skin's texture and blood flow can be enhanced. Use an exfoliating scrub or brush on the cellulite-affected areas to eliminate dead skin and increase circulation.

• Improve skin suppleness and conceal cellulite with regular moisturizing with a high-quality moisturizer. Look for moisturizers with components like hyaluronic acid, shea butter, or glycerin.

• Some topical treatments, such as creams and serums, claim to lessen the visibility of cellulite. Many of these products include caffeine, retinol, or antioxidants, all of which have been shown to increase blood flow, kickstart collagen formation, and temporarily tighten the skin. Results may be temporary and moderate, but they can still help.

• The appearance of cellulite may be lessened with regular massage, which increases blood flow and facilitates lymphatic drainage to the affected areas. Either your own hands or massage tools designed for that purpose will do the trick.

• When you dry brush, you massage your skin using a brush made of natural bristles in a circular motion. It has been shown to improve circulation and lymphatic drainage. It's important to take care when dry brushing so as not to irritate the skin.

• **Self-Tanning:** Darkening the skin with self-tanning creams can help conceal cellulite by giving the impression of a more even tone. Self-tanner works best when applied in an even layer.

• UV damage from the sun can be prevented by taking preventative measures. The skin's suppleness can be reduced by exposure to UV radiation, which can accentuate existing cellulite. Sunscreen should be used at all times when outdoors.

• Maintaining a healthy, well-rounded diet that's high in fruits, vegetables, and whole grains helps improve skin quality and may help minimize the appearance of cellulite in ways that aren't immediately apparent.

• In order to maintain healthy skin, proper hydration is essential. In order to keep skin pliable and promote a healthier appearance, proper hydration is essential.

Keep in mind that the success of skincare methods in reducing cellulite varies from person to person and that the effects tend to be short-lived. The most successful method of reducing the appearance of cellulite is to take a holistic approach to its management, which entails keeping a healthy lifestyle with good nutrition and frequent exercise. Although cellulite is a normal part of the aging process, your skin can seem younger and healthier by taking care of it generally.

CHAPTER FIVE
Cosmetic Surgery and Other Medical Procedures

Cellulite can be treated and concealed with the use of cosmetic and medical procedures. The degree to which these treatments invade patient autonomy varies widely. It's best to talk to a doctor or dermatologist about your specific situation to figure out which treatment is best for you. Common treatments for cellulite, both medical and cosmetic, include:

1. Creams and lotions sold at drugstores and supermarkets all claim to diminish the visual effects of cellulite. Common active components in such items include caffeine, retinol, and antioxidants. They may provide some relief temporarily, but their efficacy varies and their effects are usually minimal.

2. Lymphatic drainage massage is one massage technique that has been shown to temporarily increase blood flow and decrease cellulite. Excess fluid can be removed from the affected areas with the use of massage, as it stimulates lymphatic circulation.

3. Effective laser treatments for cellulite reduction include radiofrequency and ultrasound techniques. The suppleness of the skin is enhanced, fat cells are dissolved, and collagen formation is boosted. These therapies aren't intrusive, but you may need more than one session to see a difference.

4. Endermologie is a non-invasive technique that involves massaging and manipulating the skin using a mechanical instrument with rollers. The goal is to lessen the appearance of cellulite by enhancing metabolic processes like blood flow, collagen synthesis, and lymphatic drainage. Usually, a few appointments are required.

5. Subcision is a minimally invasive treatment in which a thin needle is used to cut the fibrous bands that are dragging the skin down and causing the dimpled appearance of cellulite. When compared to less intrusive methods, the effects of this surgery tend to persist longer.

6. Minimally invasive laser therapy called Cellulaze attacks cellulite at its source. Laser light is used to sever fibrous bands, melt fat, and kick-start collagen production. This treatment, when administered by a medical expert, tends to last for quite some time.

7. Dermal fillers like Sculptra, which are injected under the skin, have been shown to increase skin elasticity and minimize the appearance of cellulite by stimulating the body's natural synthesis of collagen. The effects are short-lived and will need regular upkeep.

8. Liposuction refers to a surgical technique that eliminates fat deposits. Although it may be effective in reducing the fat deposits that contribute to cellulite, it was not developed for this purpose and may not have the desired effect. Liposuction is mainly used for body reshaping.

9. Mesotherapy is a method of treating obesity and poor circulation by injecting a vitamin, mineral, and chemical solution into the skin. This non-surgical option may require more than one session.

The success rates of these treatments vary, and the benefits they provide are frequently just short-term. Furthermore, not everyone will benefit from these approaches, and some may even be harmful. Talk to a doctor about your concerns, goals, and expectations before agreeing to any treatment or surgery. In addition to these measures, a healthy lifestyle with a balanced diet and frequent exercise can aid in cellulite management.

Alternative Medicines and Home Remedies

Home remedies and natural therapies for cellulite reduction work by enhancing skin health, circulation, and muscle tone. These methods may not be as effective in reducing cellulite on their own as medical or cosmetic procedures, but they can help when used in conjunction with a healthy lifestyle. The following are some home treatments and natural therapies for cellulite:

• When you dry brush, you massage your skin using a brush made of natural bristles in a circular motion. It has been shown to increase circulation, aid lymphatic drainage, and exfoliate the skin. It's important to take care when dry brushing so as not to irritate the skin.

• Scrub your skin with coffee grounds and some healthy oil, such olive or coconut. The caffeine in coffee can temporarily tighten and tone the skin.

• Maintaining a healthy weight and promoting healthy skin can be aided by eating a balanced diet high in fruits, vegetables, whole grains, and lean proteins. It may also be helpful to limit one's consumption of sugary and processed foods.

• Drinking plenty of water can help the skin stay hydrated, which in turn makes it look fuller and less dimple-prone.

• **Exercising:** Regular cardio and weight training can help tone muscles, increase circulation, and diminish the look of cellulite.

• Some herbs, such gotu kola and horse chestnut, have been shown to promote circulation, which may in turn benefit skin health. Before starting any new herbal treatment, talk to your doctor.

• Some people find that using apple cider vinegar to their problem areas helps reduce cellulite. It's supposed to help tighten skin and make it smoother. It should be diluted with water before being applied to the skin.

• **Keep Moving:** Sedentary behavior has been linked to the development of cellulite. Take frequent breaks to stand, stretch, and walk in order to maintain some level of activity throughout the day.

• Getting adequate shut-eye is crucial to your health and the appearance of your skin. Aim for seven to nine hours of sleep per night.

• If you smoke, stopping can have a positive effect on your skin. Cigarette smoke has been shown to thin the skin and slow blood flow, both of which can amplify the look of cellulite.

• The appearance of cellulite may be lessened via regular massage, which works by increasing blood flow and facilitating lymphatic drainage to the affected areas.

- **Controlling Your Weight:** Cellulite can be reduced by keeping your weight at a healthy level. Rapid weight loss or growth might make cellulite more visible.

Keep in mind that the effectiveness of natural remedies and home treatments may vary and that improvement may be slow. It can be difficult to get rid of cellulite entirely because it is a naturally occurring condition. A holistic strategy to treating and minimizing the visibility of cellulite includes a balanced diet, regular exercise, and overall healthy lifestyle choices.

CHAPTER SIX
Promoting Body Acceptance

Creating a positive self-perception begins with fostering a constructive self-relationship. It's about loving and accepting your body as it is, regardless of social beauty standards or external pressures. Here are some things you can do and habits you may form to promote body positivity:

• Self-love entails accepting oneself as one is and realizing that one's worth is not contingent on one's physical attributes. Give yourself the same loving care that you would give a close friend or family member.

• Refuse to give in to negative self-talk or thoughts that make you feel bad about your physique. Challenge these ideas as they come up and reframe them in a more positive light. Look at what your body is capable of doing rather than dwelling on its apparent defects.

• Reduce Your Exposure to Unrealistic Beauty Standards Be aware of the media and social forces that promote unattainable beauty standards and take steps to limit your exposure to them. Don't keep up with or read posts that make you feel bad about your physique.

• Recognize that there is beauty in a variety of forms and sizes. To extend your horizons, immerse yourself in a variety of ideals of beauty.

• **Self-Care:** Make time for activities that restore your sense of well-being. For example, you could work out frequently, eat well, get plenty of sleep, and do things that make you happy.

• If you want to feel better about yourself and more confident about your body, try using positive affirmations. Keep reminding yourself of your value and specialness.

• Practice mindful eating by paying attention as you eat. Instead of following a rigorous diet, it's better to listen to your body's signals of when it's hungry and when it's full. Eat healthy foods to fuel your body, but don't deny yourself the occasional treat.

• **Clothes That Work:** Put on something that doesn't make you feel self-conscious. Avoid forcing yourself into unflattering sizes and instead opt for looks that make you feel confident.

• Get in touch with people who will cheer you on and encourage you to embrace your body as it is. Communicate your worries and hopes to them.

• Mastering the art of critical media analysis is a key component of achieving media literacy. Realize that media portrayals of people's appearances are not always accurate due to editing and retouching of photos.

• Gratitude is a practice that can help you feel better about yourself and your life. Practicing gratitude is a great way to change your frame of mind.

- Seek the counsel of a mental health expert who specializes in body image issues if you feel you need help overcoming low self-esteem or a negative perception of your physical appearance.

- Make Sure they're reasonable And Focused On Your Well-Being, Not Just Your Appearance If you have health and fitness goals, make sure they're reasonable, attainable, and focused on your well-being, not just your appearance.

- **Challenge Comparison:** Avoid comparing yourself to others, whether in real life or on social media. Keep in mind that no two people are taking the same path.

It takes time and work to build body positivity. Being patient with yourself and praising your progress at each milestone is crucial. Keep in mind that the most attractive qualities are those that come from within, like liking and accepting oneself just as one is.

Maintenance and Protection Against Cellulite

A mix of a healthy lifestyle and regular self-care routines is what it takes to prevent cellulite and keep skin healthy over time. You may not be able to entirely get rid of cellulite, but there are ways to make it less noticeable and stop it from getting worse. For long-term protection against cellulite, consider the following:

1. Eat Well and Stay Fit:

• Fruits, vegetables, whole grains, and lean meats should make up the bulk of your diet.

Reduce your use of processed foods, sugary snacks, and excess salt, all of which have been linked to increased body fat and fluid retention.

If you want your skin to look and feel its best, it's important to maintain proper hydration.

2. Doing Exercise on a Regular Basis:

• Regular exercise should consist of both cardio (walking, jogging, swimming) and strength training (weightlifting, bodyweight exercises).

Exercise can lessen the appearance of cellulite by decreasing overall body fat and increasing muscular tone.

3. Obtain and sustain a weight that is good for you. The look of cellulite may be exacerbated by rapid weight gain or decrease.

4. If you smoke, stopping can have a positive effect on your skin. Because smoking weakens the skin and decreases blood flow, it accentuates the appearance of cellulite.

5. Limit Your Sun Exposure:

• Wear sunscreen and protective gear to avoid sunburn. Sagging skin and cellulite may be the result of UV radiation damaging collagen and elastin fibers.

6. Care for Oneself:

• Dry brushing, massage, and consistent exfoliation are all great forms of self-care that may be incorporated into a beauty program. These methods have been shown to enhance circulation and smooth out the skin.

7. Dehydration of the Skin:

• Moisturizers and body creams will help your skin retain its natural moisture. Skin that is healthy and well-hydrated typically appears more even and flat.

8. Natural Health Aids: Herbal Products

• Some herbs, such as gotu kola and horse chestnut, are believed to enhance circulation and may help to better skin health. Herbal remedies and supplements should only be used after discussing their use with a qualified medical expert.

9. Reducing Stress:

• Chronic stress might lead to hormonal abnormalities that may impact the development of cellulite. Try some relaxation methods on for size, including yoga, meditation, or just taking some deep breaths.

10. Clothes Options:

• Dress in a way that makes you feel good about yourself. Don't wear clothes that are too snug, as this can cause blood flow problems.

11. Learn to Accept Yourself and Your Body:

• Cultivate a good body image by practicing self-love and body positivity. Instead than dwelling on your perceived defects, concentrate on your body's strengths and what it is capable of.

12. Help from Experts:

• Discuss medical and cosmetic procedures with a dermatologist or medical specialist if you're looking for more intense treatments or guidance for cellulite management.

Keep in mind that cellulite is a natural and typical condition that can be difficult to completely get rid of. The most efficient method of controlling and reducing cellulite's visibility is to take a holistic approach to skin health and general wellness. It's important to be kind to yourself and recognize small victories along the path.

Conclusion

Many people feel self-conscious about their looks due to cellulite, which manifests as dimpled or lumpy skin on the thighs, buttocks, and other places. Genetics, hormonal shifts, getting older, and personal choices all have a role.

Eliminating cellulite entirely may be impossible, but there are ways to make it less noticeable and boost your skin's health anyway. These measures include establishing a healthy lifestyle with a balanced diet, regular exercise, and self-care routines. Home treatments, homemade skincare products, and natural therapies can help support these initiatives.

Laser therapy, subcision, and injectable fillers are just some of the medical and cosmetic interventions that may help reduce the appearance of cellulite for those who want more dramatic results. It is essential, however, to confer with medical experts in order to ascertain the optimal strategy for achieving one's unique demands and objectives.

Body acceptance and the promotion of body positivity are also crucial. Individuals can learn to accept their bodies as they are, cellulite and all, via the cultivation of a positive self-image, the exercise of self-love, and the prioritization of general well-being.

Keep in mind that cellulite is completely normal and in no way indicative of your value or attractiveness. One's individual path to reducing cellulite and improving skin health is unique to them, but ultimately, everyone wants to be happy and healthy in their own skin.

THE END